HEALTH ASSESSMENT
A pocket guide

June M. Thompson, R.N., M.S.
Assistant Professor of Nursing,
School of Nursing, The University of Texas,
Houston, Texas

Arden C. Bowers, R.N., M.S.
Instructor, College of Nursing;
Instructor, Department of Psychiatry,
College of Medicine, Ohio State University,
Columbus, Ohio

Illustrated

The C.V. Mosby Company
St. Louis • Toronto • Princeton   1984

A TRADITION OF PUBLISHING EXCELLENCE

Editor: Barbara Ellen Norwitz
Developmental editor: Sally Adkisson

International Standard Book Number 0-8016-4936-6

Printed in the United States of America

The C. V. Mosby Company
11830 Westline Industrial Drive, St. Louis, Missouri 63146

PE/CB/CB   9 8 7 6 5 4 3 2 1   03/B/365

Contents

Part 1

TOTAL HEALTH DATA BASE

BIOGRAPHICAL DATA

1. Name
2. Age
3. Race
4. Culture
5. Address
6. Marital status
7. Children and family in home
8. Occupation
9. Means of transportation to health care facility, if pertinent
10. Description of home; size and type of community

REASON FOR VISIT

One statement that describes the reason for the patient's visit, or the chief complaint. State in the patient's own words.

PRESENT HEALTH STATUS

1. General health status of the patient in the past 1 year, 5 years, now
2. Summary of patient's current major health concerns
3. If illness is present, include (symptom analysis) history (p. 10)
   a. When was patient last well
   b. Date of problem onset
   c. Character of complaint
   d. Nature of problem onset
   e. Course of problem
   f. Patient's hunch of precipitating factors
   g. Location of problem
   h. Relation to other body symptoms, body positions, and activity
   i. Patterns of problem
   j. Efforts of patient to treat
   k. Coping ability
4. Current medications
   a. Type (prescription, over-the-counter drugs, vitamins, etc.)
   b. Prescribed by whom
   c. Amount per day
   d. Problems

CURRENT HEALTH STATISTICS

1. **Immunization status (note dates or year of last immunization)**
   a. Tetanus, diphtheria, pertussis
   b. Mumps
   c. Rubella
   d. Polio
   e. Tuberculosis tine test
   f. Influenza
2. **Allergies (describe agent and reactions)**
   a. Drugs
   b. Foods
   c. Contact substances
   d. Environmental factors
3. **Last examinations (note physician/clinic, findings, advice, and/or instructions)**
   a. Physical
   b. Dental
   c. Vision
   d. Hearing
   e. ECG
   f. Chest radiograph
   g. Pap smear (females)

PAST HEALTH STATUS

Although each of the following is asked separately, the examiner must summarize and record the data *chronologically*.

1. **Childhood illnesses:** rubeola, rubella, mumps, pertussis, scarlet fever, chickenpox, strep throat
2. **Serious or chronic illnesses:** scarlet fever, diabetes, kidney problems, hypertension, sickle cell anemia, seizure disorders, blood infections
3. **Serious accidents or injuries:** head injuries, fractures, burns, other trauma
4. **Hospitalizations:** elaborate reason for, location, primary care providers, duration
5. **Operations:** what, where, when, why, by whom
6. **Emotional health:** past problems, help sought, support persons
7. **Obstetrical history**
   a. Complete pregnancies: number, pregnancy course, postpartum course, and condition, weight, and sex of each child
   b. Incomplete pregnancies: duration, termination, circumstances (including abortions and stillbirths)
   c. Summary of complications

FAMILY HISTORY

Cancer	Retardation
Diabetes	Alcoholism
Heart disease	Endocrine diseases
Hypertension	Sickle cell anemia
Epilepsy (or seizure disorder)	Kidney disease
Emotional stresses	Unusual limitations
Mental illness	Other chronic problems

REVIEW OF PHYSIOLOGICAL SYSTEMS

The purpose of this component of the data base is to collect information about the body regions or systems and their function.

1. **General—reflect from patient's previous description of current health status**
   a. Fatigue patterns
   b. Exercise and exercise tolerance
   c. Weakness episodes
   d. Fever, sweats
   e. Frequent colds, infections, or illnesses
   f. Ability to carry out activities of daily living
2. **Nutritional**
   a. Patient's average, maximum, and minimum weights during past month, 1 year, 5 years
   b. History of weight gains or losses (time element; specific efforts to change weight)
   c. Twenty-four-hour diet recall (helpful to mail patient chart to fill in prior to visit)
   d. Current appetite
   e. Who buys, prepares food?
   f. Whom does patient normally eat with?
   g. Is patient able to afford preferred food?
   h. Does patient wear dentures? Is chewing a problem?
   i. Patient's self evaluation of nutritional status
3. **Integumentary**
   a. Skin
      (1) Skin disease or skin problems or lesions (wounds, sores, ulcers)
      (2) Skin growths, tumors, masses
      (3) Excessive dryness, sweating, odors
      (4) Pigmentation changes or discolorations
      (5) Pruritus (itching)
      (6) Texture changes
      (7) Temperature changes
   b. Hair
      (1) Changes in amount, texture, character
      (2) Alopecia (loss of hair)
      (3) Use of dyes
   c. Nails
      (1) Changes in appearance, texture
4. **Head**
   a. Headache (characteristics, including frequency, type, location, duration, care for)
   b. Past significant trauma
   c. Vertigo (dizziness)
   d. Syncope
5. **Eyes**
   a. Discharge (characteristics)
   b. History of infections, frequency, treatment
   c. Pruritus (itching)
   d. Lacrimation (excessive tearing)

e. Pain in eyeball
f. Spots (floaters)
g. Swelling around eyes
h. Cataracts, glaucoma
i. Unusual sensations or twitching
j. Vision changes (generalized or vision field)
k. Use of corrective or prosthetic devices
l. Diplopia (double vision)
m. Blurring
n. Photophobia
o. Difficulty reading
p. Interference with activities of daily living

6. **Ears**
a. Pain (characteristics)
b. Cerumen (wax)
c. Infection
d. Hearing changes (describe)
e. Use of prosthetic devices
f. Increased sensitivity to environmental noise
g. Vertigo (dizziness)
h. Ringing and cracking
i. Care habits
j. Interference with activities of daily living

7. **Nose, nasopharynx, and paranasal sinuses**
a. Discharge (characteristics)
b. Epistaxis (nosebleed)
c. Allergies
d. Pain over sinuses
e. Postnasal drip
f. Sneezing
g. General olfactory ability

8. **Mouth and throat**
a. Sore throats (characteristics)
b. Lesions of tongue or mouth (abscesses, sores, ulcers)
c. Bleeding gums
d. Hoarseness
e. Voice changes
f. Use of prosthetic devices (dentures, bridges)
g. Altered taste
h. Chewing difficulty
i. Swallowing difficulty
j. Pattern of dental hygiene

9. **Neck**
a. Node enlargement
b. Swellings, masses
c. Tenderness
d. Limitation of movement
e. Stiffness

10. **Breast**
a. Pain or tenderness
b. Swelling
c. Nipple discharge
d. Changes in nipples
e. Lumps, dimples
f. Unusual characteristics
g. Breast examination: pattern, frequency

11. **Cardiovascular**
    a. Cardiovascular
       (1) Palpitations
       (2) Heart murmur
       (3) Varicose veins
       (4) History of heart disease
       (5) Hypertension
       (6) Chest pain (character and frequency)
       (7) Shortness of breath
       (8) Orthopnea
       (9) Paroxysmal nocturnal dyspnea
    b. Peripheral vascular
       (1) Coldness, numbness
       (2) Discoloration
       (3) Peripheral edema
       (4) Intermittent claudication
12. **Respiratory**
    a. History of asthma
    b. Other breathing problems (when, precipitating factors)
    c. Sputum production
    d. Hemoptysis
    e. Chronic cough (characteristics)
    f. Shortness of breath (precipitating factors)
    g. Night sweats
    h. Wheezing or noise with breathing
13. **Hematolymphatic**
    a. Lymph node swelling
    b. Excessive bleeding or easy bruising
    c. Petechiae, ecchymoses
    d. Anemia
    e. Blood transfusions
    f. Excessive fatigue
    g. Radiation exposure
14. **Gastrointestinal**
    a. Food idiosyncrasies
    b. Change in taste
    c. Dysphagia (inability or difficulty in swallowing)
    d. Indigestion or pain (associated with eating?)
    e. Pyrosis (burning sensation in esophagus and stomach with sour eructation)
    f. Ulcer history
    g. Nausea/vomiting (time, degree, precipitating and/or associated factors)
    h. Hematemesis
    i. Jaundice
    j. Ascites
    k. Bowel habits (diarrhea/constipation)
    l. Stool characteristics
    m. Change in bowel habits
    n. Hemorrhoids (pain, bleeding, amount)
    o. Dyschezia (constipation due to habitual neglect to respond to stimulus to defecate)
    p. Use of digestive or evacuation aids (what, how often)

15. Urinary
   a. Characteristics of urine
   b. History of renal stones
   c. Hesitancy
   d. Urinary frequency (in 24-hour period)
   e. Change in stream of urination
   f. Nocturia (excessive urination at night)
   g. History of urinary tract infection, dysuria
      (painful urination, urgency, flank pain)
   h. Suprapubic pain
   i. Dribbling or incontinence
   j. Stress incontinence
   k. Polyuria (excessive excretion of urine)
   l. Oliguria (decrease in urinary output)
   m. Pyuria

16. Genital
   a. General
      (1) Lesions
      (2) Discharges
      (3) Odors
      (4) Pain, burning, pruritus (itching)
      (5) Venereal disease history
      (6) Satisfaction with sexual activity
      (7) Birth control methods practiced
      (8) Sterility
   b. Males
      (1) Prostate problems
      (2) Penis and scrotum self-examination
         practices

   c. Females
      (1) Menstrual history (age of onset, last
         menstrual period (LMP), duration,
         amount of flow, problems)
      (2) Amenorrhea (absence of menses)
      (3) Menorrhagia (excessive menstruation)
      (4) Dysmenorrhea (painful menses); treat-
         ment method
      (5) Metrorrhagia (uterine bleeding at times
         other than during menses)
      (6) Dyspareunia (pain with intercourse)

17. Musculoskeletal
   a. Muscles
      (1) Twitching
      (2) Cramping
      (3) Pain
      (4) Weakness
   b. Extremities
      (1) Deformity
      (2) Gait or coordination difficulties
      (3) Interference with activities of daily living
      (4) Walking (amount per day)
   c. Bones and joints
      (1) Joint swelling
      (2) Joint pain
      (3) Redness
      (4) Stiffness (time of day related)
      (5) Joint deformity
      (6) Noise with joint movement

    (7) Limitations of movement
    (8) Interference with activities of daily living
  d. Back
    (1) History of back injury (characteristics of problems, corrective measures)
    (2) Interference with activities of daily living

18. **Central nervous system**
  a. History of central nervous system disease
  b. Fainting episodes
  c. Seizure
    (1) Characteristics
    (2) Medications
  d. Cognitive changes
    (1) Inability to remember (recent vs. distant)
    (2) Disorientation
    (3) Phobias
    (4) Hallucinations
    (5) Interference with activities of daily living
  e. Motor-gait
    (1) Coordinated movement
    (2) Ataxia, balance problems
    (3) Paralysis (partial vs. complete)
    (4) Tic, tremor, spasm
    (5) Interference with activities of daily living
  f. Sensory
    (1) Paresthesia (patterns)
    (2) Tingling sensations
    (3) Other changes

19. **Endocrine**
  a. Diagnosis of disease states (thyroid, diabetes)
  b. Changes in skin pigmentation or texture
  c. Changes in or abnormal hair distribution
  d. Sudden or unexplained changes in height and weight
  e. Intolerance to heat or cold
  f. Exophthalmos
  g. Goiter
  h. Hormone therapy
  i. Polydipsia (↑ thirst)
  j. Polyphagia (↑ food intake)
  k. Polyuria (↑ urination)
  l. Anorexia (↓ appetite)
  m. Weakness

20. **Allergic and immunological** (Optional; use if patient indicates allergic history. Note precipitating factors in each case.)
  a. Dermatitis (inflammation or irritation of skin)
  b. Eczema
  c. Pruritus (itching)
  d. Urticaria (hives)
  e. Sneezing
  f. Vasomotor rhinitis (inflammation and swelling of mucous membrane of nose; nasal discharge)

g. Conjunctivitis (inflammation of conjunctiva)
h. Interference with activities of daily living
i. Environmental and seasonal correlation
j. Treatment techniques

21. **Does patient have any other physiological problems or disease states not specifically discussed.** If so, explore in detail (e.g., fatigue, insomnia, nervousness).

PSYCHOSOCIAL HISTORY

1. **General statement of patient's feelings about self**
2. **Feelings of satisfaction or frustration in interpersonal relationships**
   a. Home; occupants
   b. Patient's position in home relationships
   c. Most significant relationship (in and out of home)
   d. Community activities
   e. Work or school relationships
   f. Family cohesiveness patterns
3. **Activities of daily living**
   a. General description of work, leisure, and rest distribution
   b. Significant hobbies or methods of relaxation
   c. Family demands
   d. Community activities and involvement
   e. During period of day/week is patient able to accomplish all that is desired?
4. **General statement about patient's ability to cope with activities of daily living**
5. **Occupational history**
   a. Jobs held in past
   b. Current employer
   c. Educational preparation
   d. Satisfaction with present and past employment
   e. Time spent at work vs. time spent at play
6. **Recent changes or stresses in patient's life-style** (e.g., divorce, moving, new job, family illness, new baby, financial stresses)
7. **Patterns in which patient copes with situations of stress**
8. **Response to illness**
   a. Does the patient cope satisfactorily during own or others' illness?
   b. Do the patient's family and friends respond satisfactorily during periods of illness?
9. **History of psychiatric care or counseling**
10. **Feelings of anxiety or nervousness** (characteristics and coping mechanisms)
11. **Feelings of depression** (symptoms such as insomnia, crying, fearfulness, marked irritability or anger)
12. **Changes in personality, behavior, or mood**
13. **Use of medications or other techniques during times of anxiety, stress, or depression**
14. **Habits**

a. Alcohol
    (1) Kinds (beer, wine, mixed drinks)
    (2) Frequency per week
    (3) Pattern over past 5 years, 1 year
    (4) Drinking companions
    (5) Alcohol consumption increased when
        anxious or stressed?
b. Smoking
    (1) Kind (pipe, cigarette, cigar)
    (2) Amount per week/day
    (3) Pattern over past 5 years, 1 year
    (4) Smoking with others
    (5) Smoking increased when anxious or
        stressed?
    (6) Desire to quit smoking? (method,
        attempts)
c. Coffee and tea
    (1) Amount per day
    (2) Pattern over past 5 years, 1 year
    (3) Consumption increased when anxious
        or stressed?
    (4) Physiological effects
d. Other
    (1) Overeating or sporadic eating (e.g.,
        always in refrigerator, soft drink abuse,
        cookie jar syndrome)
    (2) Nail biting
    (3) Street drug usage

    (4) Nervous noneating
15. **Financial status**
    a. Sources
    b. Adequacy
    c. Recent changes in resources and expendi-
        tures

HEALTH MAINTENANCE EFFORTS

1. **General statement of patient's own physical
   fitness**
2. **Exercise** (amount, type, frequency)
3. **Dietary regulations; special efforts** (describe in
   detail)
4. **Mental health; special efforts such as group
   therapy, meditation, yoga** (describe in detail)
5. **Cultural or religious practices**
6. **Frequency of physical, dental, and vision
   health assessment**

ENVIRONMENTAL HEALTH

1. **General statement of patient's assessment of
   environmental safety and comfort**
2. **Hazards of employment** (inhalants, noise,
   heavy lifting, psychological stress, machinery)
3. **Hazards in the home** (concern about fire, stairs
   to climb, inadequate heat, open gas heaters,
   inadequate toilet facilities, concern about pest
   control, inadequate space)

4. **Hazards in neighborhood** (noise, water, and air pollution, inadequate police protection, heavy traffic on surrounding streets, isolation from neighbors, overcrowding)

5. **Community hazards** (unavailability of stores, market, laundry facilities, drugstore; no access to bus line)

Part 2

ANALYSIS OF A SYMPTOM

In addition to the health data base, the examiner must be prepared to collect in-depth information about a symptom. The following format is a data collection tool that can be used for physiological, psychological, or sociological symptoms.

CHIEF COMPLAINT

A one-sentence or brief statement using the patient's words to describe the reason for the visit. (Details about the complaint follow in the *symptom analysis* or *history of present illness section.*)

ANALYSIS APPROACH

Reconstruction from the patient's words of the body or mental processes underlying the symptom.
1. **Last time patient was entirely well**
   a. Patient may confuse onset of symptom with the first time he was *concerned* about it.
   b. Major symptom may have been preceded by other less alarming ones (e.g., fatigue) that the patient will not recall unless questioned.
2. **Date of current problem onset**
   a. Name specific date and time if possible.
   b. Inquiry about the setting at the time of onset may help establish chronology (time of day, month).
   c. How was patient feeling prior to symptom onset?
3. **Character** (describe the qualities of the problem)
   a. Move back to quoting the patient: What is the pain like? "like being stabbed"; "squeezed in a vice."
   b. Severity (does it interfere with activities of daily living?)
4. **Nature of problem onset**
   Was the onset slow? Abrupt? Noticeable to others? Use quotes if possible.
5. **Patient's hunch of precipitating factors**
   In determining aggravating or alleviating factors, word questions to avoid influencing answers. For example, angina: "What effect does walking have?" vertigo: "What happens if you move your head?"

6. **Course of problem** (did patient continue with
normal activity during episode?)
   a. Consistent
   b. Intermittent
   c. Duration
7. **Location of problem**
   a. Pinpoint
   b. Generalized, vague
   c. Radiation patterns
8. **Effect on other systems and activities**
   a. Symptoms, signs
   b. Body functions or positions
   c. Activities (body movement, exercise)
   d. Eating
9. **Patterns**
   The patient may exhibit a symptom that has
   been occurring intermittently over a period of
   time. Most previous questions have elicited
   data about the quantity and quality of *one*
   episode. This question concerns multiple episodes, identifies patterns, and provides an
   overview of chronology.
   a. *Timing*. Relate incidences to number of
   times per hour, day, week, month; inquire
   about patient's well-being during the inter-
   vals.
   b. *Duration* and quality variations. May indicate a stepping up or increase in intensity

over a period of time. ("Has it been getting
any better? Worse? Staying the same?")
   c. If there have been exacerbations or remis-
   sion, try to associate with other symptoms,
   activities, or precipitating factors.
10. **Efforts to treat**
   a. Home remedies (what and when)
   b. Body positions (e.g., bed rest)
   c. Over-the-counter medications
   d. Prescription medications and physician
   visits (give details)
11. **In-depth exploration of patient's life-style and
coping ability as related to the symptom**
   a. Pose questions to discover an association
   between daily activities and the symptom.
   (1) What mandatory activities make the
   symptom worse? For example, if stair
   climbing causes chest pain, does the
   patient have to use stairs at home or at
   work?
   (2) What activities are altered or curtailed
   because of the symptom? For example,
   if the patient complains of nocturnal
   urination, how much sleep is lost? Is
   fatigue a problem? Possible to sleep
   during the day?
   (3) Do altered activities pose a threat to the
   patient? If patient complains of dimin-

ished vision or glare, is driving hazard-
ous? Is reading part of job?
b. Pose questions that indicate an association
between patient's ability to deal with current life-style and the symptom. For example, if a mother complains of marked
fatigue, does this interfere with child-
rearing activities or management of the
home?

c. A general question such as "What does this
problem *mean* to you?" might help to summarize the previous questions. It also per-
mits the patient to voice an emotional
response to changes or problems. It may
help the examiner to grasp more fully the
impact or severity of the symptom.

Part 3

NORMAL FINDINGS OF THE PHYSICAL EXMAINATION

AREA EXAMINED	ASSESSMENT	NORMAL FINDINGS
VITAL FUNCTION ASSESSMENT	Temperature	98.6F 37C
	Blood pressure	Upper limits 140/90
	Pulse	60–90/min regular rhythm
	Height & weight	Refer to reference charts
	Vision test	
	Snellen	20/20 O.U.
	Near vision	20/20/O.U.
PATIENT IN SITTING POSITION		
EXAMINE HANDS	Surface characteristics	Smooth, warm, intact
	Characteristics of nails	Smooth, hard, no thickening
	Clubbing	No clubbing noted
	Skeletal characteristics	No deformity, tenderness, or crepitations
	Range of motion	Full ROM without pain
	Finger and hand strength	Bilaterally equal and firm grip

EXAMINE ARMS FROM HANDS TO SHOULDERS	Skin surface	Smooth, warm, intact
	Muscle strength	Bilaterally equal and strong
	Range of motion of all joints	Full ROM without pain
	Radial pulses	Bilaterally equal, regular, and strong
	Epitrochlear lymph nodes	Nodes not palpable
EXAMINE THE HEAD AND NECK	Face characteristic and symmetry	Normocephalic, symmetrical
	Skin surface characteristic	Smooth, warm, intact without lesions
	Symmetry and external characteristic of eyes and ears	Eyes and ears symmetrical
		Eye brows, lids, and lashes intact without deformity, ptosis, or lesions
		Conjunctiva, cornea, and sclera clear
		Ears have smooth auricles without lesions or discharge
	Hair characteristic	Evenly distributed; scalp without flaking, lesions, or tenderness
	Palpate facial bones and sinus	Nontender
	Evaluate TM joint clench teeth (CN V)	Joint fully mobile, no tenderness or crepitus
	Clench eyes tight, wrinkle forehead, stick tongue out, puff cheeks (CN VII, XII)	Able to perform all tasks easily, symmetrical response

AREA EXAMINED	ASSESSMENT	NORMAL FINDINGS
	Pupillary response	Pupils equal, round, react to light and accommodation (PERRLA)
	Accommodation (CN II, III)	
	Cover/uncover test	Eyes symmetrical without deviation of gaze
	Extraocular eye movements; vision field testing (CN III, IV, VI)	Both eyes show coordination; parallel movement thru the 6 cardinal fields of gaze
	Internal eye exam: reflex, disc, cup vessels, retinal surface, vitreous, maculae	Red reflex present, disc is round, cream color, margin well defined; 2:3 A/V vessel ratio; vitreous is clear; retina red/orange; no exudates or lesions; maculae 2 DD from disc
	Hearing evaluation (CN VIII)	Able to hear ticking watch or whisper at 2 feet (60 cm)
	Otoscope exam of ear canal and TM	External canal without lesions; some cerumen normal; TM intact, gray color, landmarks visible
	Rinne & Weber test (CN VIII)	Rinne: AC > BC Weber: equal lateralization
	Nasal; structure, septum position, turbinates	Nose straight, nostrils patent, mucosa pink and moist
	Evaluation of smell (CN I)	Odors properly identifiable

Mouth; gums, gingivobuccal fornices, buccal mucosa, palates	Lips moist and without lesions; mucosa, palates and gingivae pink and without lesions
Teeth; number, color, characteristic	32 teeth present, all are firmly seated and without caries or debris
Tongue; symmetry, movement, color, surface characteristic	Midline and symmetrical; pink color, no lesions
Floor of mouth; color, surface characteristics	Pink, without lesions
Oropharynx; mouth odor, uvula, tonsils, posterior pharynx	Pink color, no lesions, swelling or exudate; uvula midline; tonsils present or absent
Gag reflex (CN IX,X)	Gag reflex present
ROM of head and neck	Full and strong ROM without discomfort
Push shoulders up against examiner's hands (CN XI)	Bilaterally strong and equal muscle response
Carotid pulses	Symmetrical, strong, regular
Jugular venous distention	Not present in sitting position
Neck evaluation; thyroid, lymph nodes	Neck symmetrical, thyroid not palpable, lymph nodes nonpalpable
Light sensation evaluation to forehead, cheeks, chin (CN V)	Able to feel the light sensation at all places touched

AREA EXAMINED	ASSESSMENT	NORMAL FINDINGS
ASSESS POSTERIOR AND LATERAL CHEST	Observe and palpate symmetry and muscle development; spine position; posture	Muscles bilaterally equal; appears appropriate for age; spine has normal shape with no deformities; slight kyphosis noted; AP chest diameter < lateral chest diameter
	Observe respiration movement, quality of respirations	Diaphragmatic breathing, bilateral equal excursion
	Palpate chest wall for fremitus	Tactile fremitus bilateral equal
	Percuss for tone over chest wall	Resonant percussion tone throughout over lung fields
	Percuss CVA for tenderness	No CVA tenderness over kidneys
	Inspect, palpate, and percuss along lateral chest wall	Same as findings over posterior chest wall
	Auscultate chest walls for breath sounds	Vesicular breath sounds over most all lung fields; bilaterally equal sounds throughout
ASSESS ANTERIOR CHEST	Inspect skin color, lesions, muscular and skeletal symmetry	Skin without lesions, adequate hydration, muscles bilaterally equal
	Observe chest wall movement during respiration	Chest wall moves bilaterally equal with respirations
	Observe ease with respirations	Breathing without difficulty, posturing, or splinting

Female Breasts:

	Areolar area intact and smooth, bilaterally equal pigmentation
Evaluate breast tissue during ROM of shoulders	Breasts appear smooth, without masses, bulges, retractions, or skin lesions; striae may be present
1. arms extended over head	
2. hands behind head	
3. hands behind small of back	
4. hands pushed tightly against each other at shoulder level	
5. leans over so breasts fall away from chest wall	

Male Breasts:

| Size, symmetry, nipple discharge, enlargement | Smooth skin without masses, retractions, bulges or skin lesions |

All Patients:

Palpate anterior chest wall for stability, muscle or skeletal tenderness, or crepitations	Chest wall firm, without bulging, retractions, or asymmetry
Palpate precordium for thrills, heaves, pulsations	No thrills or heaves palpated, slight pulsation felt over chest wall
Locate PMI	PMI palpable at the 5th ICS, approximately 8 cm from the midsternal line
Palpate fremitus	Tactile fremitus bilaterally equal

AREA EXAMINED	ASSESSMENT	NORMAL FINDINGS
	Percuss anterior chest for resonance	Resonant tone percussed over most all lung fields
	Palpate all breast quadrants and areolae for lumps	Breasts firm, smooth texture throughout, without masses, bulges, retractions, or tenderness
	Palpate nipples for tissue characteristics and discharge	Nipples erect, no discharge, not tender to palpation
	Palpate lymph node areas associated with lymphatic drainage of breasts	No lymph nodes palpable
	Auscultate breath sounds of anterior chest, for rate, quality, type, and presence of adventitious sounds	Vesicular breath sounds over most all lung fields; bilaterally equal sounds throughout
	Auscultate heart (diaphragm and bell) over aortic, pulmonary, Erb's point, tricuspid, and apical areas; note rate, rhythm, location, intensity, timing, frequency, splitting, and murmurs	Rate = 60–90/min regular rhythm, S1,S2 heard in all locations; S1 louder at apex and longer in duration; S2 louder at base and shorter in duration. Splitting may be normally heard in young persons over pulmonary area; no extra sounds or murmurs
PATIENT IN LYING DOWN OR FOWLER'S POSITION		
ASSESS ANTERIOR CHEST	Inspect JVP for height seen above sternal angle	JVP at level of sternal angle when patient is elevated to 30 degrees

	Repeat breast inspection while patient is in recumbent position	Same as previously described
	Repeat breast palpation while patient is in recumbent position	Same as previously described
	Repeat palpation of anterior chest wall for cardiac movement, thrills, heaves, or pulsations	Same as previously described
	Repeat auscultation of the five areas over the heart (use diaphragm and bell)	Same as previously described
	Turn patient to the left side and repeat cardiac auscultation	Same as previously described
ASSESS ABDOMEN FROM EPIGASTRIC REGION TO PUBIS	Observe skin characteristics from pubis to epigastrium for scars, lesions, vascularity, bulges, and position and characteristics of the navel	Skin smooth, warm, well hydrated and intact; no lesions, scars, rashes, discolorations, inflammation, or bulges. Umbilicus centered, no hernia or ulceration seen
	Observe abdominal contour	Contour rounded and symmetrical
	Observe movement of abdomen, peristalsis, and pulsations	No peristalsis noted; slight pulsations may be seen above umbilicus and over aorta in thin individuals

AREA EXAMINED	ASSESSMENT	NORMAL FINDINGS
	Auscultate all quadrants of abdomen for bowel sounds bruits, and venous hum	Bowel sounds of gurgles and clicks present in all 4 quadrants: 5-30/min; no bruits or venous hums heard
	Percuss all quadrants and epigastric region of abdomen for tone	Tympanic sounds heard in all quadrants; dullness may be heard over superpubic region
	Percuss upper and lower liver borders for position and tenderness	Lower border of liver percussed at costal margin or slightly below. Upper border percussed between 5th to 7th intercostal spaces. Mid clavicular liver span is 6–12 cm. Mid sternal liver span is 4–8 cm. Percussion tone over liver is dull. Liver is nontender to percussion
	Percuss left-mid-axillary line for splenic dullness	Area of splenic dullness extends from 6th–10th ribs
	Light palpation of all four quadrants for tenderness, guarding, and masses	Abdomen relaxed and smooth; no tenderness or masses felt
	Deep palpation of all four quadrants for tenderness, guarding, and masses	May exhibit some tenderness over midline at xiphoid, over cecum, and over sigmoid colon; aorta may be palpated at epigastrium; feces may be palpated along descending colon; no masses palpated

Deep palpation of right costal margin for liver border	Liver often not palpable; may "bump" downward against fingers; liver border should be smooth and nontender
Deep palpation of left costal margin for splenic border	Spleen not normally palpable
Deep palpation of abdomen for right and left kidneys	Lower poles of kidneys may be felt in a thin individual; contour should be smooth and nontender
Evaluate abdominal reflexes with pointed instrument (evaluation of T_8–T_{12})	Abdominal muscles contract slightly; bilaterally equal response; umbilicus moves slightly toward area of stimulus
Client raises head for evaluation of flexion and strength of abdominal muscles	ROM of neck should permit chin to chest flexion; abdominal muscles are firm and prominent and permit patient to raise head easily off exam table
Light palpation of inguinal region for lymph nodes, femoral pulses, and bulges	Nodes not palpable; strong bilaterally equal femoral pulses palpated; inguinal region without bulges or tenderness
ASSESS LOWER LIMBS AND HIPS Assess feet and legs for skin integrity, vascular sufficiency, pulses, and skeletal formation of legs, feet and toes	Skin intact without lesions or dryness; limbs appear well hydrated without evidence of pallor, venous stasis, or edema; bilaterally equal and strong pulses at popliteal, dorsalis pedis, and posterior tibial positions; feet and toes without swelling or deformity; toes and feet maintain extended and straight positions

AREA EXAMINED	ASSESSMENT	NORMAL FINDINGS
	Palpate feet and lower legs for temperature, tenderness, and deformities	Legs and feet warm to touch; good capillary refill following blanching technique; no tenderness with palpation
	Perform ROM and muscle strength of hips, knees, ankles, feet, and toes	Full active ROM of all joints without limitations or discomfort
	Palpate hips for stability	Hips bilaterally symmetrical and stable; no discomfort with palpation
ASSESS GENITAL, PELVIC REGION, AND RECTUM	**Males:** inspect and palpate external genitalia, including pubic hair, penis, scrotum, testes, epididymides, and vas deferens; (Move patient to lateral knee chest position)	Pubic hair has triangular configuration with hair extending up linea alba to umbilicus Penis without lesions, induration or discharge. Scrotal contents palpated without tenderness or masses
	Inspect perianal area and anus for surface characteristics	Perianal and anal surfaces show no presence of rashes, inflammation, masses or hemorrhoids
	Palpate anus, rectum, and prostate with gloved finger; note stool characteristics when gloved finger is removed	Good sphincter tone; anal and rectal mucosa smooth and without masses; prostate palpated bilobed and firm without tenderness or enlargement; stool noted as brown and soft

Females: (position patient in lithotomy position)

Inspect and palpate external genitalia including pubic hair, labia, clitoris, urethral and vaginal orifices, perineal and perianal area, and anus

Hair distribution inverted triangular shape, no masses or lesions noted; labia, vestibule, and urethra intact without redness or tenderness; no foul odor or discharge noted; perineum intact

Insert speculum and inspect surface characteristics of vagina and cervix

Cervix midline, pink, firm, and mobile without lesions, is round or slit shape; vaginal surface rugous and moist

Remove speculum and perform bimanual palpation of vagina, cervix, uterus, and adnexa to assess form, size, and characteristics

Uterus pear shaped 5–8 cm long, fundus firm and anterior: contour smooth and nontender, freely moveable with palpation; ovaries and tubes may not be palpable; no masses or tenderness palpated

Perform vaginal-rectal examination to assess recto-vaginal septum and pouch, surface characteristics, and broad ligament

Septum smooth and firm; cul-de-sac and rectum without nodules, tenderness, or masses

Perform rectal exam to assess anal sphincter tone and surface characteristics; note stool characteristics when gloved finger is removed

Good sphinter tone; anal and rectal mucosa smooth and without masses; stool noted as brown and soft

AREA EXAMINED	ASSESSMENT	NORMAL FINDINGS
PATIENT IN SITTING POSITION		
ASSESS NEUROLOGICAL SYSTEM	Observe patient move from lying to sitting position; note use of muscles, ease of movement, and coordination	Good muscle coordination and strength; pushes off with arms and hands; balance OK; no noted limitations or weaknesses
	Test sensory function of neurological system by using sharp and dull, deep and light sensation of forehead, paranasal sinus areas; hands, lower arms, feet and lower legs	Sensations correctly interpreted as sharp or dull, and light or deep, at all areas tested
	Bilaterally test and compare vibratory sensation of bony areas of ankle, wrist, and sternum	Sense of vibration equally felt at all positions tested
	Test two-point discrimination of back of hand, thigh, and back	Can distinguish 2-point discrimination hands: 8–12 mm thigh: 60–75 mm back: 40–70 mm
	Test stereognosis or graphesthesia	Appropriate identification of object or written number

Test fine motor proprioception and cerebellar function and coordination of upper extremities by instinct; patient to do at least 2 of the following: 1. alternating pronation and supination of forearms 2. touching nose with alternating index fingers 3. rapidly alternating finger movements to thumb 4. rapid movement of index finger between nose and examiner's finger	Appropriate identification of object or written number Purposeful and bilaterally equal response to all commands; movements done quickly and with precision
Test and bilaterally compare fine motor function and coordination of lower extremities by instructing patient to run heel down tibia of opposite leg	Purposeful and bilaterally equal response; movements done quickly and with precision
Alternately crossing legs over knee	Purposeful and bilaterally equal response
Test and bilaterally compare deep tendon reflexes including; biceps, triceps, brachioradialis, patellar, and achilles tendons	Deep tendon reflexes (DTR) intact, bilaterally equal, quick brisk response

AREA EXAMINED	ASSESSMENT	NORMAL FINDINGS
PATIENT IN STANDING POSITION		
MALE SCROTUM AND HERNIA EVALUATION	Palpate scrotum and inguinal regions for characteristics and hernia	Scrotum palpated without tenderness or masses; all contents freely moveable and smooth; no bulges felt with hernia evaluation; triangular slit opening of inguinal ring may or may not admit examiner's finger
ASSESS NEUROLOGICAL AND MUSCULOSKELETAL SYSTEM	Assess gait	Gait smooth, coordinated, rhythmic; walks with ease, arms extended to sides, stands erect
	Observe and palpate spine as patient stands and bends forward to touch toes	Spine straight, iliac crests of equal heights, shoulders of equal heights; convexity of thoracic spine
	Stabilize patient at waist and evaluate hyperextension, lateral bending, and rotation of upper trunk	ROM with ease in all directions; no discomfort or dizziness
	Assess proprioception and cerebellar and motor function by using at least two of the following: 1. Romberg test (eyes closed) 2. walking straight heel-toe formation	Able to follow directions during all techniques; maintains upright posture with no assistance; balance is maintained throughout

3. stand on one foot and then
   the other (eyes closed)
4. hop in place on one foot and
   then the other
5. perform knee bends

Part 4

HISTORY AND PHYSICAL EXAMINATION WRITE-UP

DOCUMENTATION FORMAT

1. **Subjective data base**
   a. Biographical data
   b. Reason for visit
   c. Present health state
   d. Current health statistics: immunizations, allergies, last examination
   e. Past health status: childhood illnesses, serious or chronic illnesses, serious accidents or injuries, hospitalizations, operations, emotional health, obstetrical health
   f. Family history
   g. Review of physiological systems: general, nutritional, integumentary, head, eyes, ears, nose, mouth, neck, breast, cardiovascular, respiratory, hematolymphatic, gastrointestinal, urinary, genital, musculoskeletal, central nervous system, endocrine, and allergic and immunological
   h. Psychological history: general status, response to illness
   i. Social history: significant others, occupational history, educational level, activities of daily living, habits, financial status
   j. Health maintenance efforts: maintenance of self health, health care patterns
   k. Environmental health: general assessment, employment, home, neighborhood, community

2. **Physical assessment**
   a. Vital statistics: height, weight, temperature, pulse, blood pressure (both arms, lying, sitting, standing)
   b. General statement of appearance
   c. Mental health
   d. Integumentary: skin, nails, body hair
   e. Head and neck: scalp, hair, face, neck, lymph nodes, thyroid, trachea, sinuses

f. Nose: patency, surface characteristics
g. Mouth, pharynx: oral cavity characteristics,
    teeth, tongue, voice, tonsillar area and
    posterior pharynx
h. Ear and auditory: external ear, canal, TM
    characteristics, hearing, Rinne and Weber
    tests
i. Eye and visual: external eye characteristics,
    vision, eye movement, funduscopy
j. Thorax and lungs: thorax characteristics,
    breathing pattern and rate, percussion tone,
    auscultatory characteristics
k. Cardiovascular: all pulses, blood pressure,
    extremity circulation, precordium character-
    istics, heart sounds
l. Breast: surface characteristics, areolae and
    nipples, palpation characteristics, lymphatic
    assessment, breast self-examination assess-
    ment
m. Abdominal, rectal: contour, surface charac-
    teristics, bowel sounds, percussion tones,
    palpation characteristics, liver and spleen,
    bladder, kidney characteristics, CVA tender-
    ness, hernias, rectal examination findings
n. Genital
    (1) Female: external genitalia characteristics,
        internal—cervical, vagina, uterus,
        adnexa characteristics
    (2) Male: external genitalia characteristics,
        palpation characteristics of penis and
        scrotum, inguinal hernia evaluation
o. Musculoskeletal: muscular development and
    strength, skeletal and joint characteristics
    and symmetry, range of motion
p. Neurological: orientation, intactness of CN
    1 to XII, coordination of fine and gross
    motor movements and gait, sensory evalua-
    tion, reflexes
3. **Risk profile:** Those items from the patient's
    history and physical assessment which might
    indicate risk to the overall health state. These
    are potential problems. *Examples* that may be
    considered risk for some patients are detailed in
    the data base in Chapter I.
4. **Problem list.** The problem list should be a
    synthesis of those items which are currently
    identified as stresses for the patient. The
    stresses may be physiological, sociological,
    psychological, or a combination of these. The
    problems are those items which reduce the
    patient's overall level of health. Once the prob-
    lems are listed and assigned a priority, it can
    then be decided which are within the exam-
    iner's scope of practice to handle and which
    must be referred.
       It is important for the examiner to cluster

subjective and objective data to describe problems. The following unrelated examples demonstrate a holistic approach to problem identification.

a. Weight gain: 18 pounds in past year; exercise limited to game of tennis twice a month; expresses desire to diet but needs direction

b. Short of breath when walking up more than one flight of stairs; moderate edema below midcalf bilaterally; fine rales in lower bases bilaterally

c. Limited range of motion in right shoulder interferes with activities of daily living, dressing, preparing meals

d. Cataracts bilaterally; interfere with reading and driving at night

e. BP 180/120 (right arm) lying, 172/112 (right arm) sitting; retinal A-V ratio appears to be 2/4; arteriolar narrowing

f. Periodic slight urinary incontinence since birth of child 3 years ago; cystocele noted on vaginal examination

g. Complaints of LLQ discomfort for 6 months; cyclic with menses; ↑ discomfort at ovulation time and just prior to menses; thickening in left adnexa area; ↑ tenderness with palpation of left adnexa area; menses regular; pinpoint tenderness on deep palpation in LLQ

h. Smokes one pack of cigarettes a day for past 15 years; deep nonproductive cough for past 5 years, becoming worse; ↑ breathing difficulty when climbing more than one flight of stairs; ↓ breath sounds on right; bilateral rales or rhonchi in base of lungs; slight clearing with cough

i. Death of spouse 2 months ago; since then ↑ periods of depression, 10-pound weight loss. ↓ desire to maintain own health state

Part 5

ANATOMICAL GUIDELINES

HEAD AND NECK

Anatomical landmarks of lateral head and neck

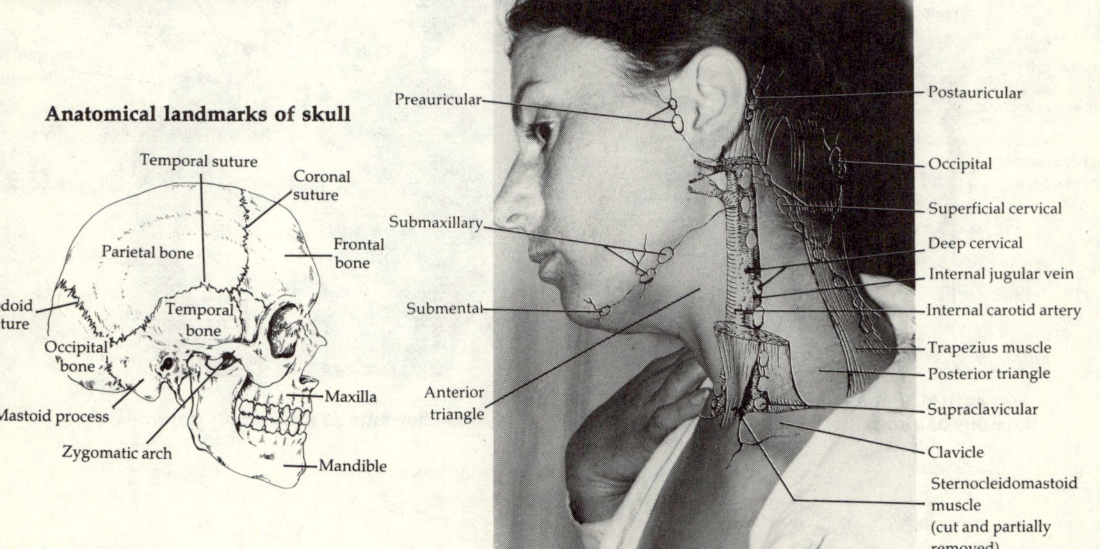

Anatomical landmarks of skull

EYES

Anatomical landmarks of anterior neck

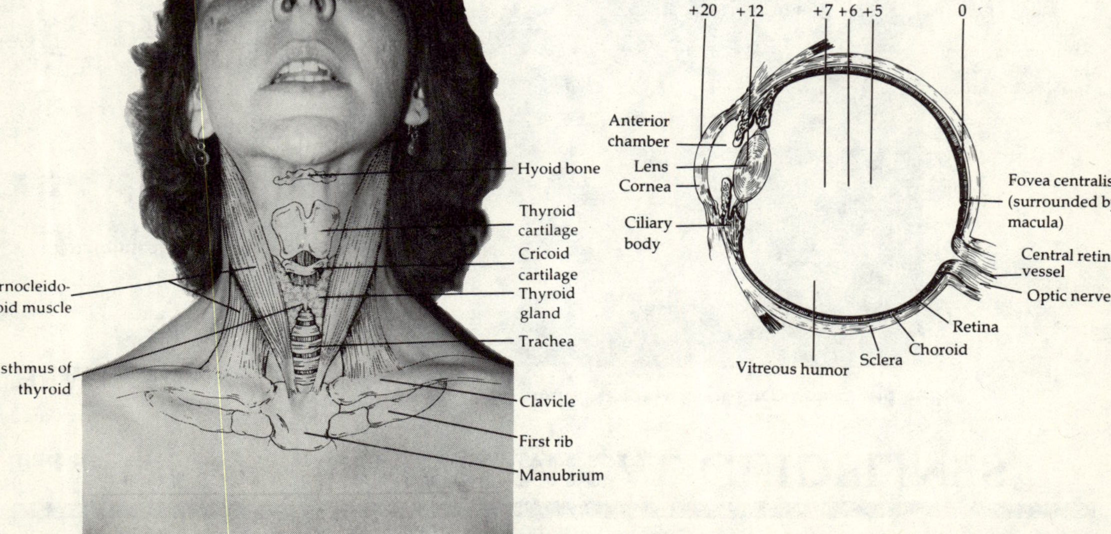

Longitudinal cross-section of eye showing focused ophthalmoscope lens settings

EARS

Six cardinal fields of gaze

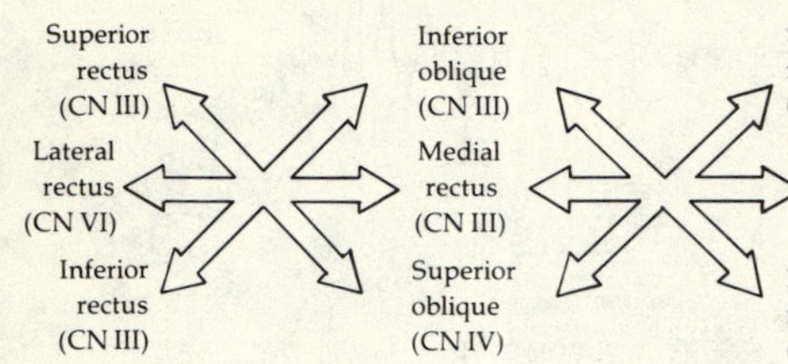

Optic disc landmarks

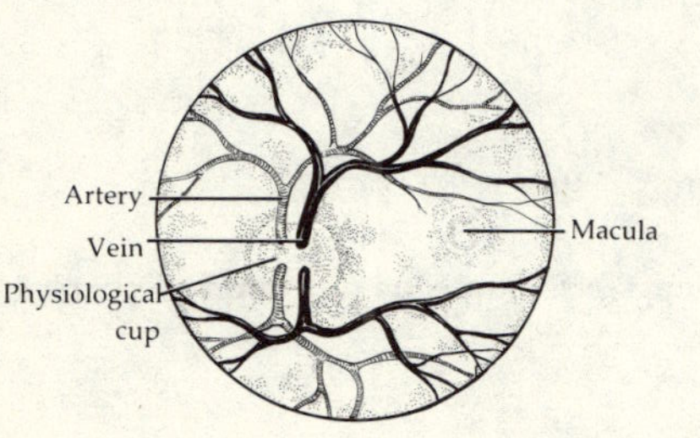

Tympanic membrane landmarks

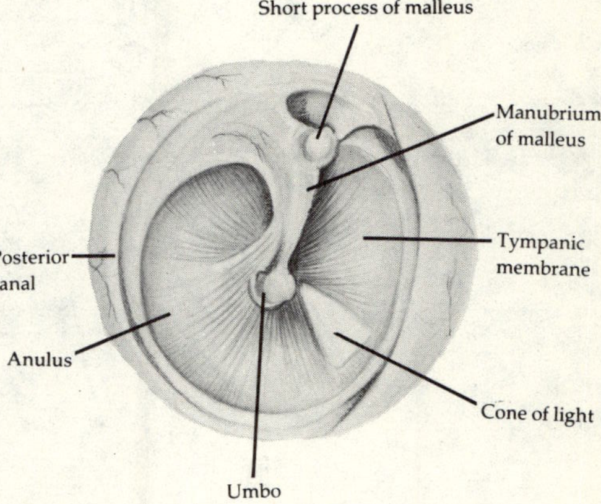

MOUTH

Average age of eruption and shedding of deciduous teeth

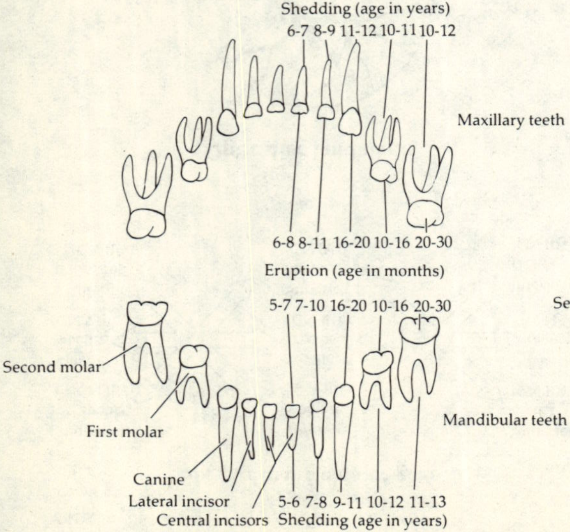

Average age of eruption of permanent teeth

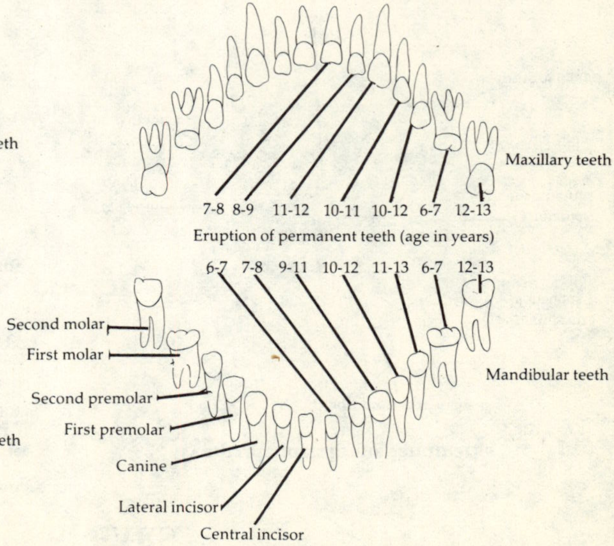

THORAX AND LUNGS

Topographical landmarks of thorax

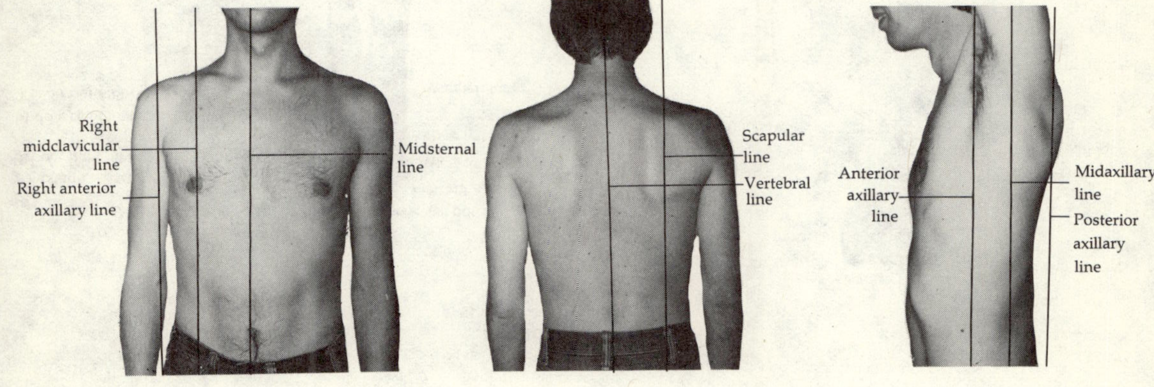

Anatomy of thorax

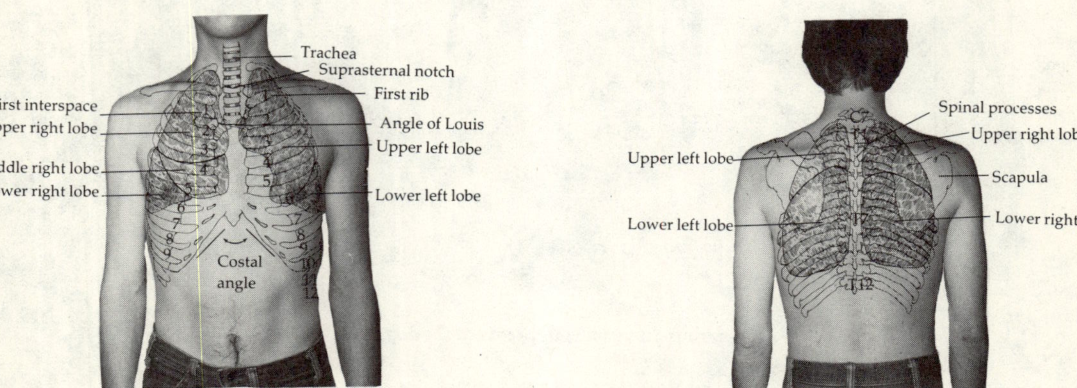

Percussion tones of thorax

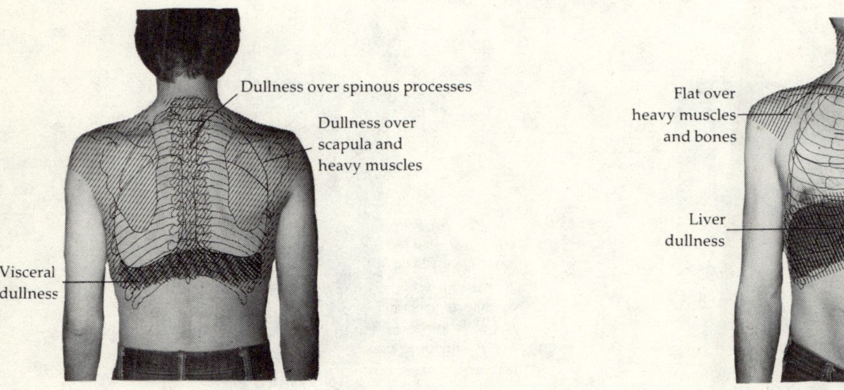

Breath sounds over lung fields

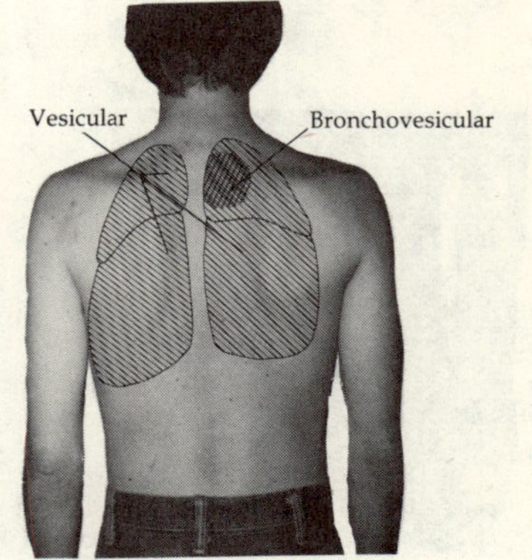

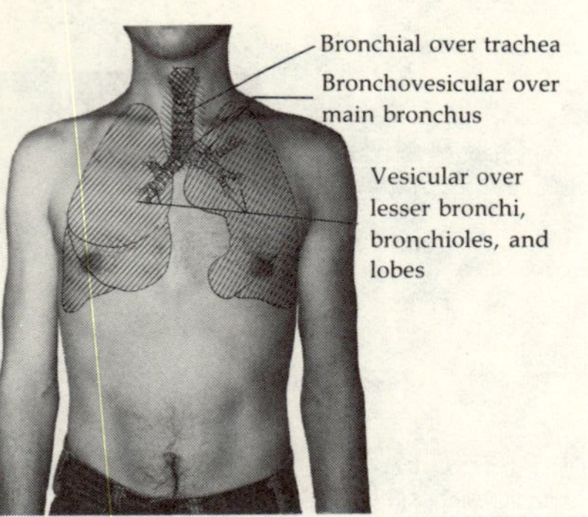

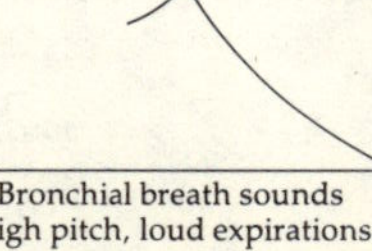

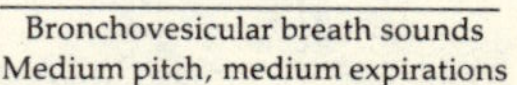

Vesicular breath sounds
Low pitch, soft expirations

Bronchial breath sounds
High pitch, loud expirations

Bronchovesicular breath sounds
Medium pitch, medium expirations

Adventitious breath sounds

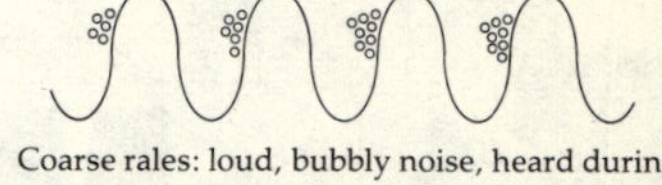

Adventitous sounds, including rales and fine rales, high-pitched crackling sound, heard toward end of inspiration; indicates inflammation or congestion

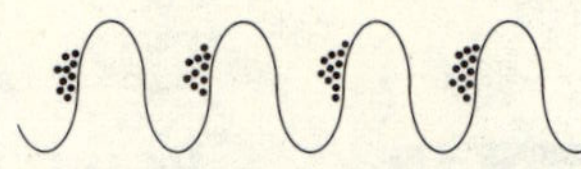

Medium rales: lower, more moist sound, heard about halfway through inspiration
Found in clients with pneumonia or pulmonary edema (not cleared by cough)

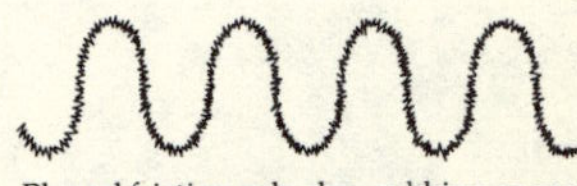

Coarse rales: loud, bubbly noise, heard during inspiration
Found in clients with pneumonia (not cleared by cough)

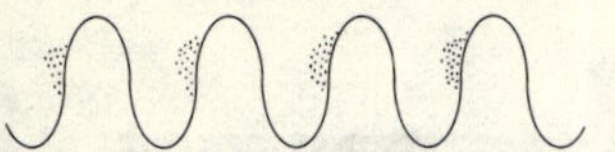

Rhonchi: small airway noise
Sibilant rhonchi (wheeze): musical noise like squeak
May occur during inspiration or expiration, but usually louder during expiration

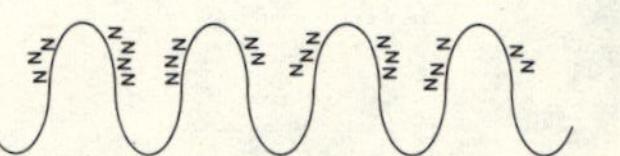

Sonorous rhonchi (wheeze): low, loud, coarse sound like snore; may occur at any point of inspiration or expiration; usually means obstruction of trachea or large bronchi (coughing may clear sound)

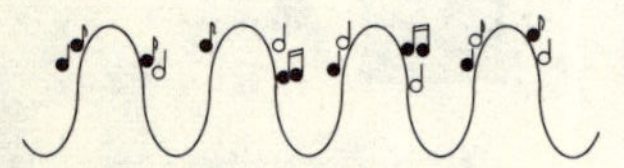

Pleural friction rub: dry, rubbing or grating sound usually due to inflammation of pleural surfaces: heard throughout inspiration and expiration: loudest over lower anterior lateral surface

CARDIOVASCULAR

Palpation areas for cardiac examination

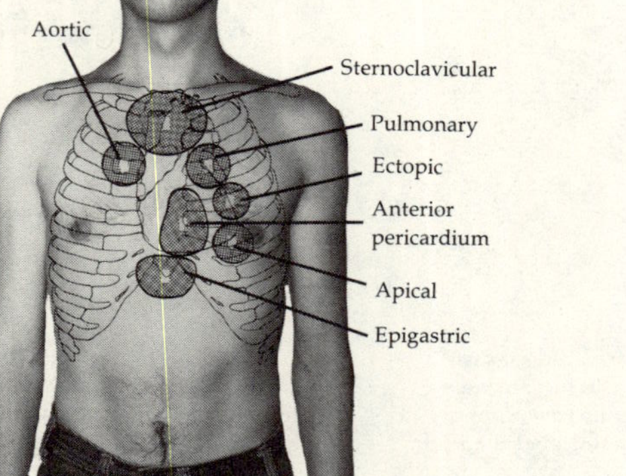

Anatomical and auscultatory valve areas

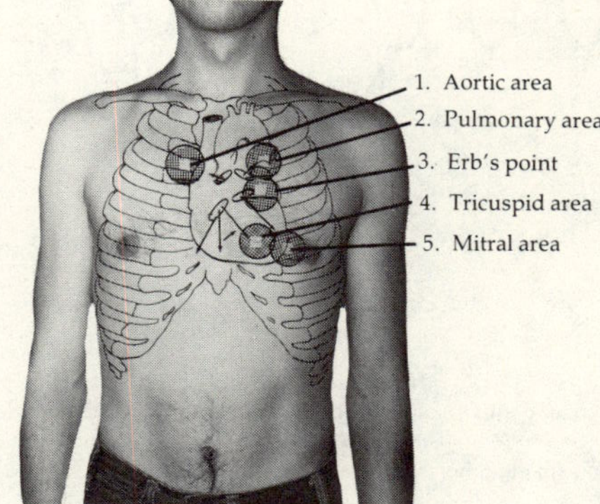

BREAST

Lymphatic drainage of breast

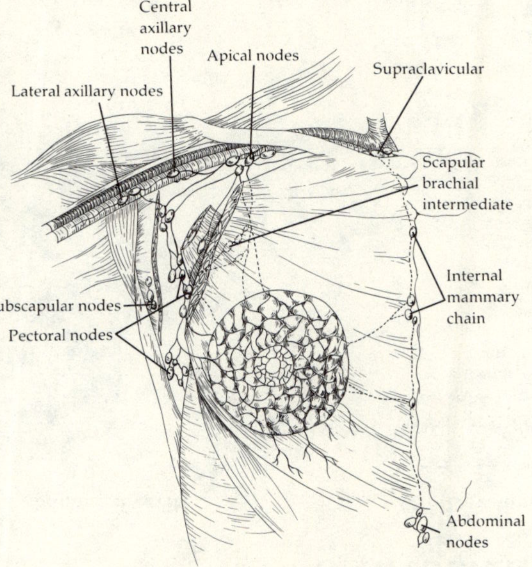

ABDOMEN

Major structures of abdominal cavity

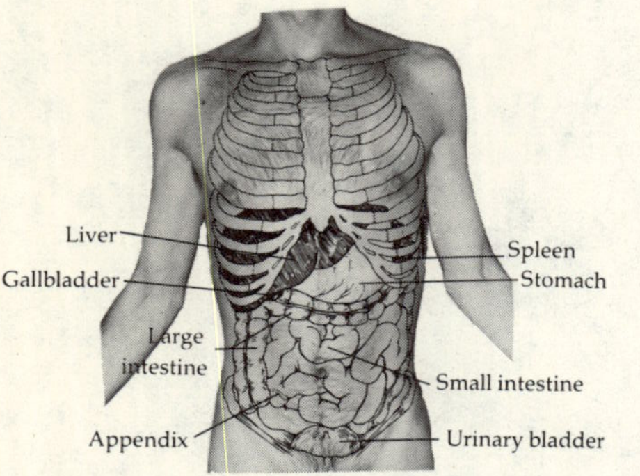

GENITOURINARY

Development in females

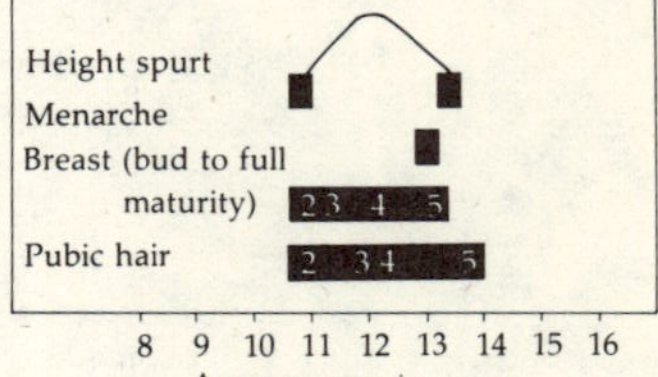

Development in males

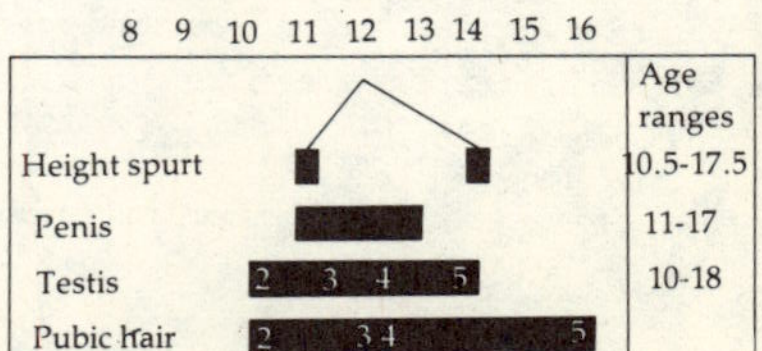

MUSCULOSKELETAL

Musculoskeletal functional assessment

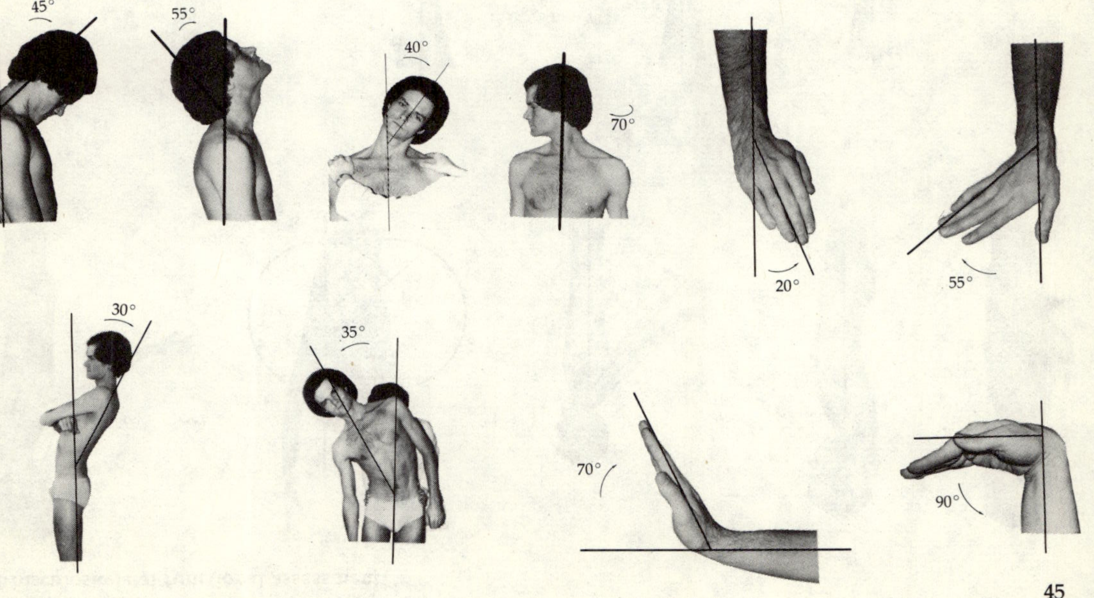

Musculoskeletal functional assessment

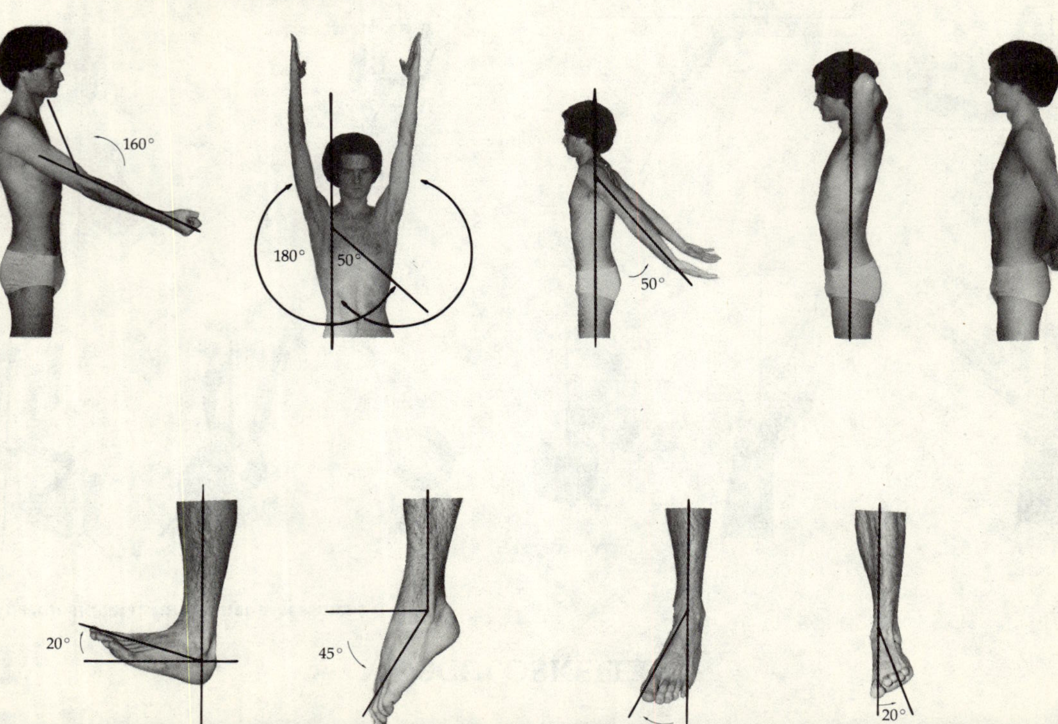

Musculoskeletal functional assessment

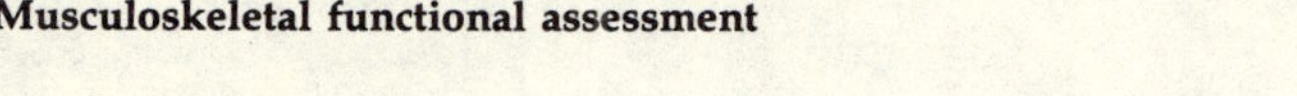
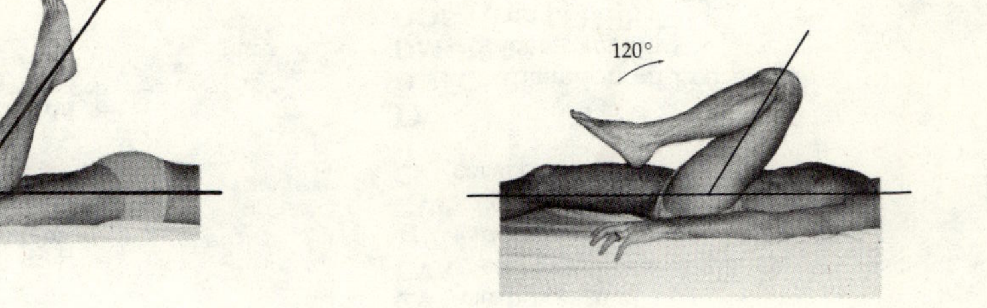

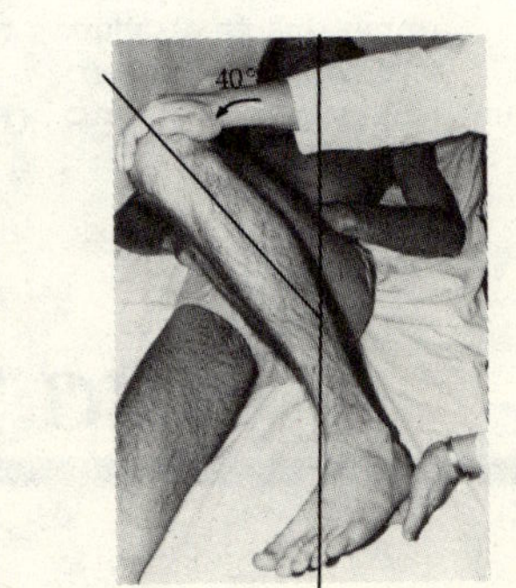

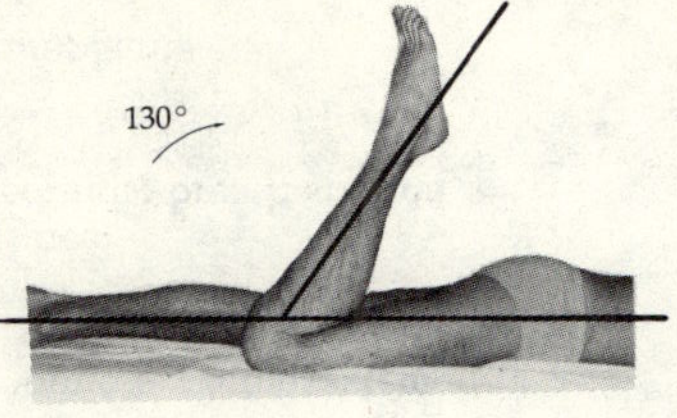

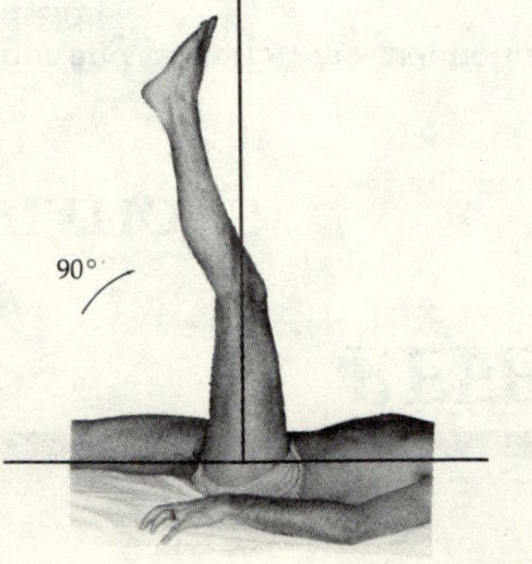

Part 6

REFERENCE DATA

ABBREVIATIONS

A
A & P anterior and posterior; auscultation and
percussion
A & W alive and well
abd abdomen; abdominal
AJ ankle jerk
AK above knee
ANS autonomic nervous system

B
BK below knee
BS bowel sounds; breath sounds

C
CC chief complaint

CHD childhood disease; congenital heart disease;
coronary heart disease
CHF congestive heart failure
CNS central nervous system
COPD chronic obstructive pulmonary disease
CV cardiovascular
CVA costovertebral angle; cerebrovascular acci-
dent
CVP central venous pressure
Cx cervix

D
D & C dilatation and curettage
DM diabetes mellitus
DOB date of birth
Dx diagnosis

E

ECG, EKG   electrocardiogram; electrocardiograph
EENT   eye, ear, nose, and throat
ENT   ear, nose, and throat
EOM   extraocular movement

F

FB   foreign body
FH   family history
Fx   fracture

G

GB   gallbladder
GU   genitourinary
GYN   gynecological

H

HOPI   history of present illness
Hx   history

I

IOP   intraocular pressure

J

JVP   jugular venous pressure

L

lat   lateral

L

LCM   left costal margin
LLQ   left lower quadrant (abdomen)
LMP   last menstrual period
LS   lumbosacral
LSB   left sternal border
LUL   left upper lobe (lung)
LUQ   left upper quadrant (abdomen)

M

MSL   midsternal line

N

N & T   nose and throat
N & V   nausea and vomiting
NSR   normal sinus rhythm

O

OD   right eye
OM   otitis media
OS   left eye
OU   both eyes

P

P & A   percussion and auscultation
PE   physical examination
PERRLA   pupils equal, round, react to light and
accommodation
PI   present illness

PID pelvic inflammatory disease
PMH past medical history
PMI point of maximum impulse; point of maximum intensity
PVC premature ventricular contraction

R
RCM right costal margin
REM rapid eye movement
RLQ right lower quadrant (abdomen)
ROM range of motion
RUQ right upper quadrant (abdomen)

S
SQ subcutaneous

T
T & A tonsillectomy and adenoidectomy
TPR temperature, pulse, and respiration

U
URI upper respiratory infection
UTI urinary tract infection

CONVERSION TABLES

Length

In.	cm.	cm.	In.
1	0.5	1	0.4
2	0.9	2	0.8
4	1.8	3	1.2
6	2.7	4	1.6
8	3.6	5	2.0
10	4.5	6	2.4
20	9.1	8	3.1
30	13.6	10	3.9
40	18.2	20	7.9
50	22.7	30	11.8
60	27.3	40	15.7
70	31.8	50	19.7
80	36.4	60	23.6
90	40.9	70	27.6
100	45.4	80	31.5
150	66.2	90	35.4
200	90.8	100	39.4

1 inch =
2.54 cm.

1 cm =
0.3937 inch

Weight

lb.	Kg.	Kg.	lb.
1	0.5	1	2.2
2	0.9	2	4.4
4	1.8	3	6.6
6	2.7	4	8.8
8	3.6	5	11.0
10	4.5	6	13.2
20	9.1	8	17.6
30	13.6	10	22
40	18.2	20	44
50	22.7	30	66
60	27.3	40	88
70	31.8	50	110
80	36.4	60	132
90	40.9	70	154
100	45.4	80	176
150	66.2	90	198
200	90.8	100	220

1 lb. =
0.454 Kg.

1 Kg. =
2.204 lb.

HEIGHT AND WEIGHT TABLES FOR ADULTS

Desirable weights for men
(according to frame, ages 25–59)

HEIGHT (in shoes)†		SMALL FRAME	MEDIUM FRAME	LARGE FRAME
Feet	Inches			
5	2	128–134	131–141	138–150
5	3	130–136	133–143	140–153
5	4	132–138	135–145	142–156
5	5	134–140	137–148	144–160
5	6	136–142	139–151	146–164
5	7	138–145	142–154	149–168
5	8	140–148	145–157	152–172
5	9	142–151	148–160	155–176
5	10	144–154	151–163	158–180
5	11	146–157	154–166	161–184
6	0	149–160	157–170	164–188
6	1	152–164	160–174	168–192
6	2	155–168	164–178	172–197
6	3	158–172	167–182	176–202
6	4	162–176	171–187	181–207

Data from: Build study, 1979, Society of Actuaries and Association of Life Insurance Medical Directors of America, 1980. Copyright 1983 Metropolitan Life Insurance Company.
*Weight in pounds (in indoor clothing weighing 5 pounds).
†Shoes with 1-inch heels.

Desirable weights for women
(according to frame, ages 25–59)

HEIGHT (in shoes)†		SMALL FRAME	MEDIUM FRAME	LARGE FRAME
Feet	Inches			
4	10	102–111	109–121	118–131
4	11	103–113	111–123	120–134
5	0	104–114	113–126	122–137
5	1	106–118	115–129	125–140
5	2	108–121	118–132	128–143
5	3	111–123	121–135	131–147
5	4	114–127	124–138	134–151
5	5	117–130	127–141	137–155
5	6	120–133	130–144	140–159
5	7	123–136	133–147	143–163
5	8	126–139	136–150	146–167
5	9	129–142	139–153	149–170
5	10	132–145	142–156	152–173
5	11	135–148	145–159	155–176
6	0	138–151	148–162	158–179

Data from: Build study, 1979, Society of Actuaries and Association of Life Insurance Medical Directors of America, 1980. Copyright 1983 Metropolitan Life Insurance Company.
*Weight in pounds (in indoor clothing weighing 5 pounds).
†Shoes with 1-inch heels.

BOYS: BIRTH TO 36 MONTHS—PHYSICAL GROWTH, NCHS PERCENTILES

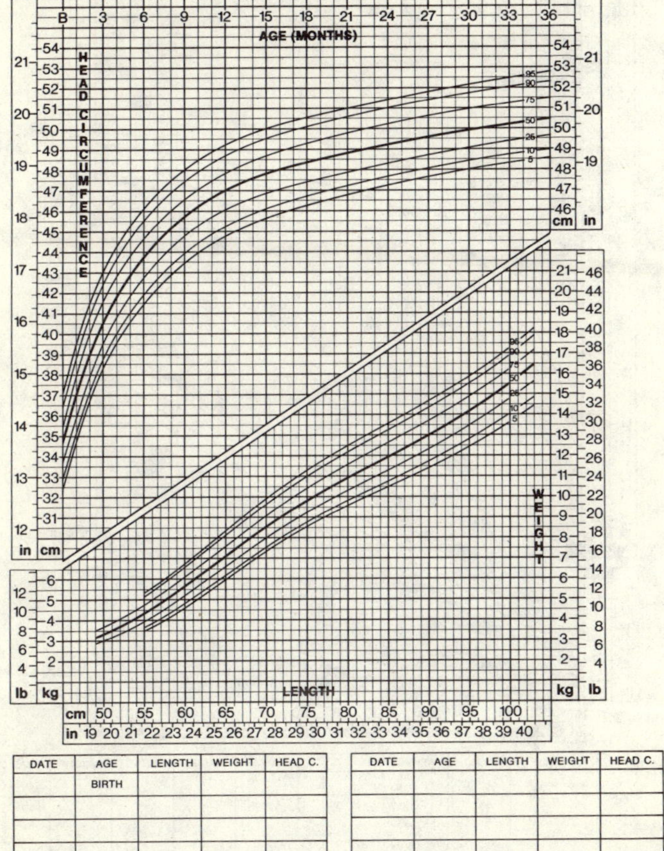

DATE	AGE	LENGTH	WEIGHT	HEAD C.
	BIRTH			

DATE	AGE	LENGTH	WEIGHT	HEAD C.

(Adapted from Hamill, P.V.V., and others: Physical growth: National Center for Health Statistics percentiles, Am. J. Clin. Nutr. 32:607–629, 1979. Data from the Fels Research Institute, Wright State University School of Medicine, Yellow Springs, Ohio. Provided as a service of Ross Laboratories, 1980.)

GIRLS: BIRTH TO 36 MONTHS—PHYSICAL GROWTH, NCHS PERCENTILES

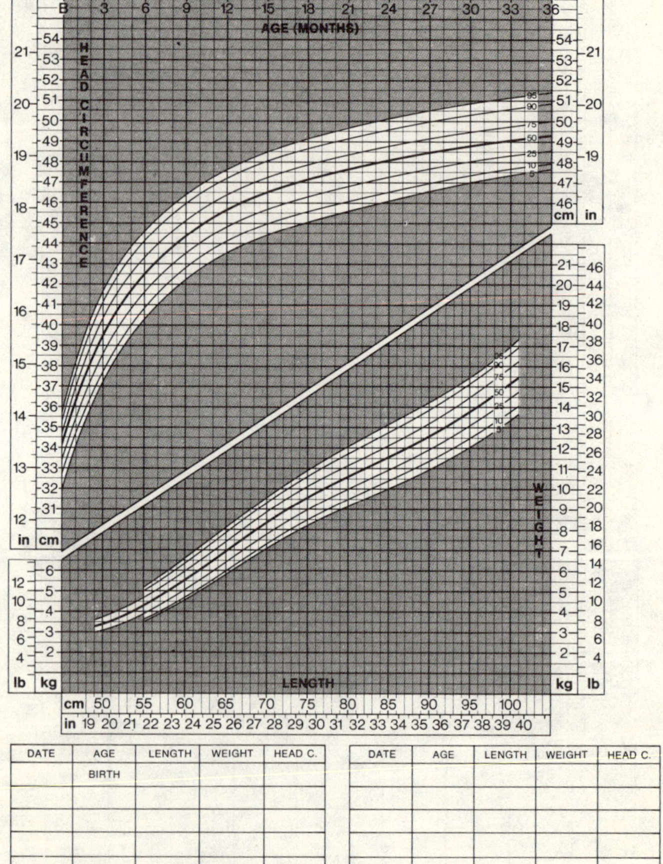

DATE	AGE	LENGTH	WEIGHT	HEAD C.
	BIRTH			

DATE	AGE	LENGTH	WEIGHT	HEAD C.

(Adapted from Hamill, P.V.V., and others: Physical growth: National Center for Health Statistics percentiles, Am. J. Clin. Nutr. 32:607–629, 1979. Data from the Fels Research Institute, Wright State University School of Medicine, Yellow Springs, Ohio. Provided as a service of Ross Laboratories, 1980.)

BOYS: 2 TO 18 YEARS—PHYSICAL GROWTH, NCHS PERCENTILES

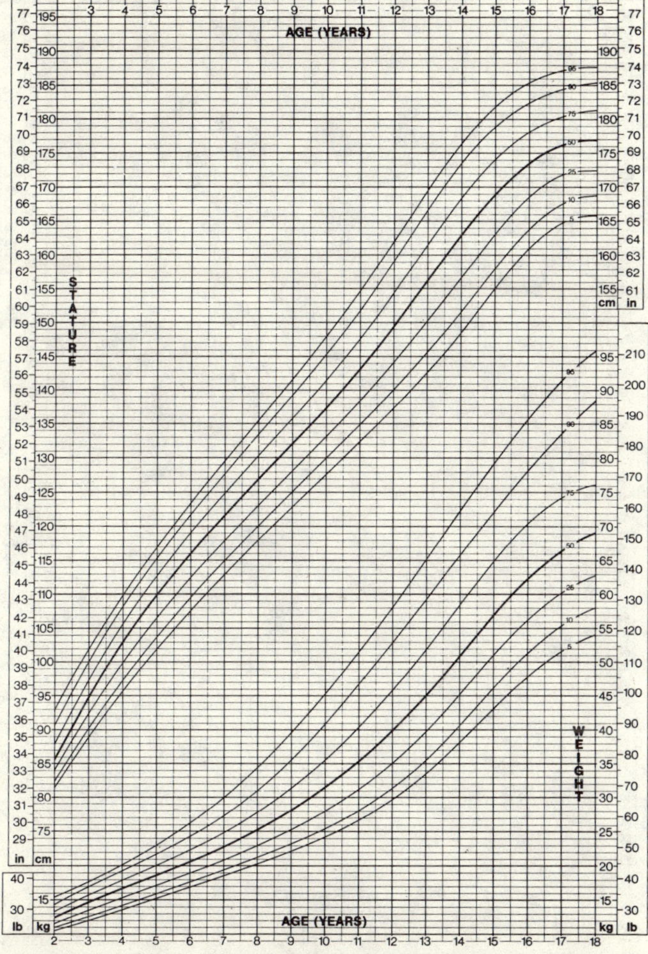

(Adapted from Hamill, P.V.V., and others: Physical growth: National Center for Health Statistics percentiles, Am. J. Clin. Nutr. 32:607–629, 1979. Data from the National Center for Health Statistics [NCHS], Hyattsville, Md. Provided as a service of Ross Laboratories, 1980.)

GIRLS: 2 TO 18 YEARS—PHYSICAL GROWTH, NCHS PERCENTILES

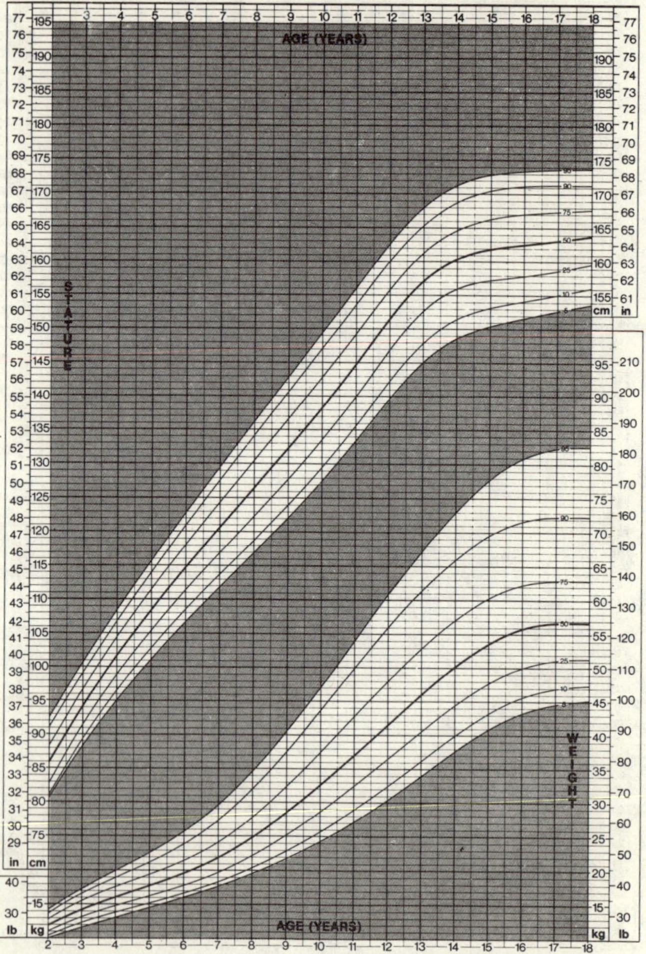

(Adapted from Hamill, P.V.V., and others: Physical growth: National Center for Health Statistics percentiles, Am. J. Clin. Nutr. 32:607–629, 1979. Data from the National Center for Health Statistics [NCHS], Hyattsville, Md. Provided as a service of Ross Laboratories, 1980.)

ROSENBAUM POCKET VISION SCREENER

95

874

2843

638 ЕШЭ ХОО

8745 ЭШШ ОХО

6 3 9 2 5   ШЕЭ   X O X

4 2 8 3 6 5   ШЕШ   O X O

3 7 4 2 5 8   ЭШЭ   X X O

9 3 7 8 2 6   ШШЕ   X O O

4 2 8 7 3 9   ЕШШ   O O X

distance equivalent	Point	Jaeger
20/800		
20/400		
20/200	26	16
20/100	14	10
20/70	10	7
20/50	8	5
20/40	6	3
20/30	5	2
20/25	4	1
20/20	3	1+

METRIC 1 2 3 4 5 6 7 8 9 10 11 12 13 14

INCHES 1 2 3 4 5

Card is held in good light 14 inches from eye. Record vision for each eye separately with and without glasses. Presbyopic patients should read thru bifocal segment. Check myopes with glasses only.

DESIGN COURTESY J. G. ROSENBAUM, M.D.

NOTES

NOTES

NOTES